The Metamorphosis of a Butterfly

A Journey of Rebirth, Hope and Transformation

by Joy Hadji Alliy

Typesetting and Printing:

Mkuki na Nyota Publishers Ltd

P. O. Box 4246

Dar es Salaam, Tanzania

www.mkukinanyota.com

To
Asha Mtindo
and
Ross Methven

*"When you focus on the journey, you will be blessed with
guardian angels to direct your path."*

- Lailah Gifty Akita.

CONTENTS

Introduction..1

THE BREAKDOWN...3

The Machine 5

Crash 13

Repair 17

RECOVERY 27

Denial and Despair..29

Rehabilitation..37

Relationships...41

Hope...46

ACCEPTANCE 52

Mental Battles 54

Shame..60

Empathy 66

Compassion...71

BRUISED NOT BROKEN 79

Regaining Control 81

Learning To Cope 85

Close Companion 88

Positive Language 92

Peace and Tranquility 96

Holidays 100

Epilogue 104

Introduction

This is my honest and true account of an ischaemic stroke that I suffered on 27 September 2020, and my experience as a stroke survivor. Any feelings that I experienced at any point in time were my own and were not influenced by any third party. My psychiatrist encouraged me to be completely open about my feelings as part of my therapy, and as a way to encourage and hopefully inspire others.

I had an ischaemic stroke, which is caused by a blockage in an artery that supplies blood to the brain. The blockage reduces the blood flow and oxygen to the brain, leading to damage or death of brain cells.

In order to make sense of the emotions that I was experiencing I had the opportunity to speak with a few stroke survivors as well as family members of survivors.

Every stroke survivor's experience is different but we all share a common need which many people fail to understand; the need to be supported emotionally as much as possible and be surrounded by empathetic people, the need to have our feelings acknowledged no matter how ludicrous or childish they might appear to be, and the need to be heard.

Our behaviours may become erratic or change completely during the recovery period. Therefore, we sometimes do not act like normal people, nor control how we feel.

This journey has made me realize who you can trust and rely on in dark times, and that we don't have to try to be kind. We just have to stop being unkind.

I hope that my story will help carers and family members to have a better understanding of stroke survivors, raise awareness of the condition and help reduce the stigma attached to the mental health element of stroke recovery.

PART I

THE BREAKDOWN

CHAPTER ONE

The Machine

"We can choose to be perfect and admired or to be real and loved."

- Glennon Doyle Melton

I started my legal career when I was 25 and joined what was one of the biggest law firms in Tanzania at the time. I hated litigation and going to court but was in my element whenever I worked on transactional projects that involved the government, the oil and gas sector and project finance.

There were two lawyers at the firm that I looked up to as mentors. They inspired me and helped shape my career. These were Dr Wilbert Kapinga and Lucy Henry Sondo. Dr Kapinga is a brilliant man; very intelligent, a natural leader, a rainmaker and a great teacher. He believed in me from day one and always encouraged me to take on challenging assignments to further my legal skills. He and the founder and managing partner Mr Mkono were impressed with my ability to quickly manage government projects in the oil and gas sector which were new areas to the firm at the time.

I worked on building up my confidence and both Mr Mkono and Dr Kapinga came to depend on me as I could be trusted to get the work done independently. One thing I wish I had learnt from him was his ability to stay calm under pressure. The building could be going up in smoke, but Dr Kapinga woud just slowly emerge from his office wondering what all the commotion was about.

Lucy Sondo stood tall, exuded an incredible amount of confidence, and was incredibly driven. A senior associate at the time, Lucy already exhibited many leadership attributes, making her partnership material. Her legal prowess, strong work ethic and ability to charm clients, yet still let them know not to cross the line, used to leave me thinking "Damn, I want to be her when I grow up".

The legal profession can be incredibly competitive and ruthless, and yet Lucy still found time to mentor the junior associates and help promote the wellbeing of those around her. She was always incredibly warm and friendly, with a very cheeky sense of humour.

The early years were a struggle for me, working long hours and fighting to be recognised as an equal in a society and industry where women are viewed as second class citizens. I spent almost nine years working at the firm and the hard work paid off. I made junior partner in the seventh year and got my first mention in the Chambers Global Guide, which ranks top law firms and lawyers in over 200 countries. Dr Kapinga was delighted and extremely proud of my achievement.

I had been working nonstop up until this point and my ambition, drive and perfectionism had forced me to operate in robot mode. I thought I was invincible. However, I started to notice a change in my performance. I was exhausted, struggling to make it into work every day I desperately needed a break. Leaving the firm was one of the most difficult choices I had to make. I was leaving behind my work family, and my mentor who had become like a second father. But it had to be done. I was suffering from burnout, although this did not even exist as a concept back then.

I always wanted to become a dually qualified lawyer so I took my opportunity during my hiatus to go to law school in the UK and received a postgraduate diploma in legal studies from the Oxford Institute of Legal Studies, a program that was jointly run by Oxford University and Oxford Brookes University.

After two years away from work and trying for months to get a training contract from a UK firm, I decided to come back home and was ready to return to the corporate world. I assured myself that this time it was going to be different. I was going to look after myself and avoid burnout. The problem was that I had always set very high expectations of myself. Even when I was in primary school, I always made sure I had top grades and went crying to my mother one day when I got a B.

Upon my return to Tanzania I joined a much smaller firm, hoping for better working hours and a more balanced life. Old habits die hard though, and I soon fell back into the same routine of working long hours and not looking after myself. I continued to prosper and shine at the new firm, getting my second mention in Chambers, a win that I quietly celebrated.

Things were looking up. I was a promising young lawyer with an enviable salary and a good life. Towards the end of 2014, however, that came to a grinding halt when my mother was diagnosed with pancreatic cancer. This happened in the middle of a high-level government transaction that I had been working on daily for over two years. My mother died 4 months after her diagnosis and her passing hit me like a ton of bricks. I felt like my heart

7

had been ripped into a thousand pieces.

Being a very private person I refused to cry in front of people during the days leading up to the funeral. I went to the gym one day to let off some steam and thought I was alone in the spinning room. I started crying so hard and didn't realise that someone else had come into the room, and was wondering why I was so upset. It has now been over 7 years and I am still mourning her loss. I never properly allowed myself to grieve, putting on a brave face for others, and chose to hide behind mountains of work, instead of processing her passing and getting closure.

After a year of passive mourning and feeling very lost, I decided it was time to move on from the firm. The decision to leave was made easy when I suffered a serious panic attack at work. I quit my job the very next day and instead of taking some time off, I set up my own law firm less than one month later.

Setting up a law firm in Tanzania was no easy feat. I had limited savings but was conscious that I had to make a good impression both in terms of the office location and the quality of lawyers.

The first three months were spent working from home on my dining table. Later, my father offered me some office space in a building that he owned. The space was still dust and concrete when I moved in with my first employee. My father carpeted the space and we found some old furniture to use. When the firm began earning money I bought some locally made furniture and the place looked more appealing.

I couldn't afford to hire an experienced lawyer so my first employee was a single mother who was a university graduate. I trained her for many years and invested in her by paying for her to go to law school.

I prefer to work with people who are street smart and hard working rather than graduates who know nothing about the real world. So my next employee was a young lady who 'only' had a high school certificate but boy was she good. She learned the ropes very quickly and even helped the interns with their work.

I hired a number of male graduates but was disappointed with their attitude. They didn't respect me as their boss or their fellow colleagues. I decided not to renew their contracts and make it very clear to the rest of the team that I did not tolerate any form of discrimination based on gender or tribalism.

I chose to operate as a sole proprietor, and for the next 5 years my life was a never ending rollercoaster.

In the second year of practice two gentlemen from a South African law firm came to see me, and made an offer to merge with my firm. The financial compensation was enticing given the fact my savings were dwindling as I had not paid myself a salary for two years. However I had committed myself to see the venture through even if it were to fail. I had set up my own firm as I had become tired of being accountable to others and working crazy hours. I wanted to be my own boss and make my own decisions for a change. I respectfully declined their offer.

I found out a year later that Dr Kapinga had become the managing partner of the South African firm. Once again he tried to entice me and my team to merge with them and as much as I had missed working with Dr Kapinga my answer was the same. If my firm failed and everything went horribly wrong, I could still hold my head up high and say that I had tried.

And so I continued hustling to bring in new business, chasing clients for unpaid bills, arguing with suppliers over their inflated invoices, battling with the tax author ity's exaggerated assessments, dealing with employee dramas, the list went on and on.

I was elated when I appeared in Chambers again in the firm's first year. It was validation that I was on the right track, so I vowed to work even harder the following year. This meant imposing very high expectations on my team. Everything had to be near perfect and when they were not able to deliver I took on their workload instead of learning to delegate properly. Every year, whilst I revelled in my ranking, I kept pushing harder than the previous year, determined to prove wrong all the naysayers who doubted I could do it alone.

When the Covid pandemic hit Tanzania around the end of March 2020 I worried like every other business owner whether the firm would survive. We were months away from completing our fifth year and had been working very hard to build the firm's reputation.

Lady luck was on our side and we were soon overwhelmed with work. I was home alone as the Tanzanian airspace was closed off and Ross, my life partner, was stuck in Edinburgh which was under lockdown. I found myself working up to 11 pm on most days and that was when I first started experiencing dizzy spells. In the beginning, they were so bad that I couldn't work more than an hour without triggering one which lasted around twenty minutes. I managed to control the dizziness with anti-vertigo medication and soldiered on.

When we went back to the office running training sessions for my team. I encouraged them to utilize their legal skills as much as possible and learn to think independently because one day I might not be around. They probably thought I was being dramatic when I said that.

Two months later, when Ross had arrived in Dar and had gone to meet friends, I lost my vision for a split second whilst watching television. The same thing happened again another evening when we were both at home. I made a mental note to book an appointment with the opticians to get my eyes checked. The last time I lost my vision was when I was in my pool with AJ, my six-year-old nephew. I found out later from my neurologist that the dizzy spells and temporary loss of vision were transient ischemic attacks (TIAs), also known as mini strokes.

CHAPTER TWO

Crash

"Take care of your body. It's the only place you have to live."

- Jim Roh

My law firm held its fifth anniversary in September 2020 and I had a small party to mark the occasion. I gave a speech which I ended with the following quote from Benjamin Button:

"It's never too late to become who you want to be. I hope you live a life that you're proud of, and if you find that you're not, I hope you have the strength to start over."

One week later I was in hospital I had had an ischaemic stroke. A blood clot on the left side of my brain had affected my speech and the right side of my body.

Ross and I were supposed to go on a boat trip the day the stroke happened. We had both been working very hard in the weeks leading up to the anniversary, so when a good friend of ours offered us the use of his boat, we thought what better way to celebrate the occasion than to go to one of the islands nearby and treat ourselves to some champagne and lobster on the beach. As the days got closer, for some strange reason I no longer felt like going. Part of it was due to my fear of boats and the open water, but something else kept bothering me, making me want to postpone the trip.

My sister Lulu and AJ had come to visit on the day leading up to the stroke and we went for a swim. While in the water I lost my vision for a split second but didn't want to scare my nephew, so I sat on the edge of the pool and helped him with his swimming technique.

The rest of the day was uneventful. I went to get my hair done at the local salon where we chatted about how overrated weddings were becoming these days. I met up with Ross and a friend for a drink afterwards at a water front bar across the street from the salon. We went to a supermarket to buy a coolbox for the champagne and, as it was getting late by the time we got home, we ordered a takeaway and went to bed around 11 pm.

I woke up at 4 am to go to the bathroom and flipped on the light switch. I looked at myself in the mirror and didn't recognise the person staring back at me. I tried to make a sound but I didn't make any sense. "You're having a bad dream," I told myself. "Go back to bed and everything will be okay in the morning." Little did I realise how dramatically my life would change the next day.

Ross woke me at 8 am so we could get ready for the boat trip. He called out to me several times, and when he lifted the sheet off me, he immediately noticed something was wrong. I was talking gibberish and the right side of my body was very weak.

The next thing I remember was Ross somehow managing to get me out of bed, grab the car keys and we were out the door. I could see from the corner of my eyes the day watchman staring at us in disbelief.

Ross called Lulu and she met us at the nearby medical facility. Having lost my mother to pancreatic cancer 7 years ago, my sister had unknowingly taken on an additional role in her absence. I watched her looking down at me as I lay on the clinic bed, desperately trying to hold back her tears. Although we were born three years and three days apart, we had always been extremely close, despite her ruining my Rick Astley tape back in the 90s. We used to pretend we were twins and always got up to no good, including one time when we got back home late from a night out, and she made me climb over a 3-metre gate to open it as the night watchman was nowhere to be seen.

At the medical centre the nurses took my vitals and watched over me whilst we waited for the on-call doctor to arrive. After what felt like an eternity, with still no sign of the doctor, the nurses suggested we go to one of the main hospitals.

I had always been a backseat driver whenever I got in the car with Ross. However on this occasion I ignored him honking and weaving through Sunday morning traffic like a madman. Sitting in the back of the car in my sister's arms I was asking myself over and over again what went wrong. I was a very healthy 42-year-old woman with the body of a twenty-something-year-old. I was very careful about what I ate and went into my body. I didn't smoke or consume copious amounts of alcohol and had been kickboxing since 2004.

CHAPTER THREE

Repair

"In Japan broken objects are often repaired with gold. The flaw is seen as a unique piece of the object's history, which adds to its beauty. Consider this when you feel broken."

- anonymous.

We arrived at the emergency room and I was immediately wheeled into one of the treatment bays, where I was attended to by an ER doctor and team of nurses. I tried desperately to answer their questions and was frustrated that I couldn't respond quickly enough. After checking my vitals again, the doctor decided to send me up for an MRI scan to check for any blood clots and swelling. As I was weak all down the right side the right side of my body, my mouth had deviated to one side and I had difficulty talking, they were confident that I had suffered a stroke. Lulu reminded me a few weeks later why she was so distraught at the hospital our mother had had a stroke shortly before she died.

Whilst the doctors and nurses were busy attending to me, Lulu was trying to get hold of my insurance details. We quickly learnt the hard way that without adequate medical insurance or cash to pay for treatment, you might not get proper medical care. My father had signed the family up with one of the insurance companies, so I was covered. I found out later on when I was recovering, that some insurance plans have maximum financial limits on the coverage for in and out patient treatments. Once you have reached that limit, you have to cover your own medical expenses.

As we were getting ready to go up to the radiology department I briefly saw my youngest brother Mohammed and my brother in law Araf. I kept saying to them over and over that I didn't know what had happened.

My sister was allowed to accompany me to the radiology room, and as we were about to leave I mustered all the energy I had and uttered a faint "I love you" to Ross. I left him with tears welling in his eyes and went into the lift.

We arrived in the radiology room and panic immediately set in. I hated confined spaces and the last time I had an MRI scan I felt like I was trapped in a coffin. I decided that the only way I was going to get through this was to block all of my emotions. No matter how painful a procedure was, I would try to control my feelings as much as I could.

A young lady emerged from the other side of the screened room and introduced herself. Given her young age, Lulu started panicking and demanded to see her supervisor. After being assured multiple times that the lady was a very capable radiographer, Lulu calmed down.

I was injected with a tracer which hurt like hell but would allow the radiographer to get a good reading of the blood clot and brain swelling. After wrapping me up in a tight blanket and securing the sides with plastic clamps, I was wheeled into the machine. I noticed that the design of the machine had changed since the last time I had a scan. It did not feel as claustrophobic and we were done in no time.

Back in the emergency unit we waited for the paperwork to be processed before I could be admitted, and my sister had to pay a small fortune as a deposit for my care. I was a bit apprehensive about being admitted and sharing a room with a stranger. Coronavirus remained a concern, and as I have asthma I had been extremely cautious in recent months. The hospital assured me that I would have my own room in a facility called the Pavilion. Once the hospital was satisfied we would be able to cover the bills, I was transferred into another stretcher bed and wheeled up to the Pavilion with Lulu and Ross in tow.

The Pavilion was located on the fifth floor and consisted of 15 self-contained rooms with large flat screen TVs and balcony views of the ocean. The rooms could easily pass as a 4-star hotel in Tanzania if you replaced the hospital beds and railed bathrooms with king sized beds, toilet amenities, slippers and bathrobes. There was a sofa which converted into a bed, which meant that Ross could stay with me. It was my home for the next 6 days, during which time the doctors carried out further tests to ascertain what caused the stroke and continued to work on reducing the swelling on my brain.

It was after 2pm by the time I arrived in my room and I was starting to feel hungry. A woman from the catering department appeared and suggested I have kingfish with mashed potatoes. 2 hours later the food arrived with some undercooked broccoli which I found impossible to eat and the fish was full of bones. A doctor who had been doing her rounds came in and gave the catering lady a stern talking to. My jaw muscles were very weak after the stroke and I was in no shape to eat solid foods.

The medics appeared shortly with a long plastic tube and some lubricating gel. "We are going to have to put in a feeding tube so the food can go directly into your stomach" she explained. I looked over at Ross with a look of sheer panic. I had seen on TV how coronavirus tests were done where they shoved long swabs up your nose and that always freaked me out. "I've had a feeding tube up my nose before," said Ross trying to downplay it all. "It's a bit uncomfortable but it will all be over in seconds." After hesitating for some minutes I knew I couldn't prolong the process any longer, so I sat back very still and closed my eyes as the doctor inserted about 40 cm of tubing up my nose and down my throat. Soon afterwards I started producing an insane amount of saliva every few minutes. This went on throughout my first night and didn't slow down until the end of the second day.

We still hadn't told my father what had happened to me. He was upcountry with my other brother Mbwana to help him with the construction of his house. We had to find a gentle way to break the news to a 77-year-old man.

My sister called and told him he had to come back to Dar immediately as I was in the hospital having some tests. My father assumed it all had to do with the fact that I wasn't eating properly. Truth be told, aside from missing lunches whenever I was busy at work, I always made very hearty and nutritious meals in the evenings and on weekends which he never saw me eating. My thin frame had more to do with having more kickboxing classes and not upping my calorie intake.

I kept getting up every so often, armed with lots of tissues to catch my never-ending salivations, wanting to walk up and down in the corridor with either Ross or Mohamed. I was later told that I was still able to walk because I was running on adrenaline and probably still in denial about the stroke.

I was feeling anxious about what I would say to my father when I saw him. He arrived in Dar es Salaam the next day and drove straight to the hospital. Lulu and Ross sat him down outside my room at the small waiting area and explained to him what happened.

By this time the nurses had already connected some IV lines filled with medicine to my arm, and a feeding bag that went into the tube in my nose, so I was stuck in bed. My father came into the room and sat by my bed. He held my arm tightly and kept repeating "you will be okay". I couldn't look him in the eye as I was afraid I would cry, so I nodded my head and tried to be brave for both of us.

He stayed for a while, not saying much to me but recounting to Lulu and Ross his trip back to Dar and the number of times he and the driver had been stopped by the traffic police. It was getting late and my father had to go home to break his fast, so he left me to rest and promised to come back in the morning.

I have seen my father cry on three occasions. The first time was when Lulu and I were little and watched the Champ with him. He cried in the scene when Jon Voight wins the boxing match and dies shortly afterwards, leaving his son weeping over his body. The second time was when his mother passed away. The third time was when my sister and brothers met him at the airport on his return from India. He wept openly in front of his friends, who tried to console him, as we waited for our mother's body to be removed from the aeroplane. I am not sure what state he was in when he was alone in his bedroom that evening.

I tried to sleep that evening but it was impossible, with nurses coming in every couple of hours to change a line or take my blood pressure. I refused to use a bedpan as I wanted to have at least some control over my bathroom visits. This didn't go so well the first couple of days. It would take the nurses a good ten minutes to come when we called for them and by the time they finished unhooking my feeding bag and medications, I barely made it to the bathroom and ended up wetting myself a few times.

Being a modest person who would never change clothes in front of others in the gym, despite going to an all-girls school for six years, I found the idea of being bathed by a nurse very intrusive. To make matters worse, I started my period and was presented with an industrial size sanitary towel by one of the nurses.

Luckily Lulu remembered what she had to wear after giving birth to my nephew and disappeared for an hour. She came back with what appeared to be a pack of adult diapers and whisked me off to change. "How fetching. These are quite comfortable," I said to Lulu. "I could get used to them." "We will have to get you some more granny pants first" she replied. "Not those thonged matching sets that we found in your underwear drawer." I still have some leftover diapers tucked away in one of my bathroom shelves to remind me of the experience.

Around midday on day 3 my sister told me I had a visitor outside. Even though young children were not allowed on the floor, my nephew insisted on seeing Tee (short for auntie). He always looked up to me ever since he was very small, I doted on him like he was my own and we were extremely close. How could I let him see me in such a state?

I stood a few metres away from him, trying to contain myself and not to cry. He held on to his father's hand and stared at me. "He doesn't recognise me", I thought to myself. Ashamed and overcome with emotion, I motioned for Lulu to take me back to my room.

She could tell I was emotionally distraught and asked if I would like to see

Dr Kapinga and Lucy Sondo. Dr Kapinga was shocked when he heard the news and got in touch with Lucy right away. He told her to put on a nice dress as he was going to take her to visit somebody at the hospital, keeping her in the dark until they arrived.

Lucy had suffered a stroke two years prior and had made a full recovery. If there was that anybody that could lift my spirits, it was her. Before letting them in, Lulu told me to be brave and not let them see me cry. "What happened, Joy", asked Lucy in her deep warm voice. I immediately felt at ease in her presence. "Don't worry", she kept telling me. "I had a stroke and two operations and look at me now". Her stroke happened just as she was getting ready to start a board meeting. Her body gave up after many years of being pushed to the limit running her firm, being a board member for countless companies and looking after her family. She survived the stroke even though she was in a coma for three weeks. I felt comforted knowing that the same neurologist that had operated on her, Dr Philip Adebayo, was in charge of my case.

I had visited Lucy at her law firm once she was back on her feet, and she advised me not to take things too seriously, and to try to enjoy life. Unfortunately, I didn't heed her warning as I was too busy trying to prove myself to the world with my constant striving for perfection.

Dr Kapinga avoided my gaze and stared at his phone. I had known this man for eighteen years and I had never seen him like this. He was always jolly, cracking jokes and regaling us with funny stories of cases he had attended, or transactions he had worked on.

Sensing the awkwardness in the room, Lucy turned to Dr Kapinga and said to him jokingly "It is your fault that we both had strokes, you made us work so hard." "I can't help it if you are both perfectionists," he replied.

This was true. Throughout the eighteen years that I had known her, I had tried to emulate her attributes and worked twice as hard for recognition and to maintain a strong personality.

Before leaving, Lucy said a short prayer, wishing me a speedy recovery, and reassured me again that I would recover in no time. I lay there quietly for a minute after they left, reflecting on the conversation. While I was encouraged by their visit, a huge part of me felt like I had let them down. Their involvement in my professional career had compelled me to pay it forward, by mentoring and supporting the professional development of other lawyers, and I wasn't even half way through playing my part.

The remainder of the days at the hospital was spent undergoing physiotherapy and further tests to determine the cause of the stroke. I watched my nutritional feed bag trickle into my body at a snail's pace while Lulu and Ross wolfed down pancakes for breakfast every day. Good thing I have strong will power and didn't ask for a blended version to be inserted into my feeding tube.

Dr Adebayo came to check on my progress every day and reported that the swelling around the brain was smaller than they thought. The test results for MRI scan (brain), CI scan (head), ECHO, carotid doppler, thyroid and hepatitis, came back normal, as did the coronavirus and antibody tests. Lulu and Ross asked the doctor a bunch of questions and he was surprised I had none. How could I when I refused to accept that I had a stroke? I had also ceded all control to the doctors, Lulu and Ross and let them make all decisions.

Dr Adebayo was keen for me to be discharged as soon as I was stable since he believed that patients' recovery quickened when they were back in their own homes. He told us he hadn't seen his family back in Nigeria for over a year, and would therefore not be able to see me for my first consultation. I would be seeing a visiting neurologist, Dr Eric Aris.

The nurses started feeding some yoghurt through my mouth, to slowly wean me off the feeding tube. On one occasion when a nurse was feeding me, I burst into tears out of nowhere and the nurse asked me what was wrong. I told them I was so grateful that Ross found me when I had the stroke and he had been by my side ever since. I had always been wary of men, having been burnt on multiple occasions, and wasn't sure he would stick around after the stroke. The nurse turned to me and told me not to cry. All the nurses had seen how attentive and caring he was. She told me to thank God for bringing him into my life, because if it had been another man, he would have done a runner by now.

Discharge day finally arrived and I was ready to hit the road. The feeding tube was removed and a friendly dietician Rozina Ratansi brought me a meal plan which consisted of a lot of blended food, fruits, vegetables, fruit smoothies and at least two cups of milk or yoghurt every day. She had lots of great ideas on how we could make the meals tasty and I was looking forward to trying them out. I was not weighed once during my stay at the hospital, and she had assumed for meal plan purposes that I weighed 50 kg. We realised during my first out patient consultation a week later, that my weight had dropped to 45 kgs when I was in the hospital.

My prescription which consisted of blood thinners, mood enhancers and sedatives arrived, and after thanking all of the nurses and orderlies at the Pavilion, I was ready to resume my new life.

PART II

RECOVERY

CHAPTER FOUR

Denial andDespair

"Denial is the shock absorber for the soul. It protects usuntil we are equipped to cope with reality."

- C. S. Lewis

We arrived home and the familiar turquoise walls of my living room, which had a calming effect every time I walked into my apartment, had no impact on my mood. I sat down on the sofa to take stock of what had happened and I turned to Lulu. "There is something wrong with me," I said in a barely audible voice. My vocal cords were weak and I couldn't string a sentence together without running out of breath. "I don't feel anything, only sadness and anger." "Even when you see AJ?", she asked even though she already knew the answer. "I had noticed that you're not your usual self. Don't worry, the mood enhancers will kick in soon".

Even though I was barely out of the hospital I was already thinking about work. There were some projects that I had been working on which needed my attention along with some tax bills coming up. I was torn between keeping the firm going and asking my team to step up or close it down for a while. I quickly realised I was in no shape to run anything, let alone take care of myself. I was having trouble remembering things, I forgot the alphabet and found it difficult to spell simple words. To make matters worse, I had forgotten the passwords to my laptop and phones, so I could not even turn on my "out of office" notification.

I soon managed to log onto my work email account after scrambling around looking for passwords hidden in note- books, and left a cryptic out-of-office message: "Please be advised that Joy is out of the office until further notice and does not have access to emails". I thought writing "I'm recovering from a stroke" would be too much. I gave my team the option of staying on and looking after the firm on their own or to close shop, and they assured me that they would manage. The firm's bank accounts were temporarily frozen and only allowed to accept upcoming funds, and I reluctantly handed over control of the firm's expenses to my father.

The first week home was challenging as there was no manual on how to care for a stroke patient that we could follow. I knew I couldn't drink water in case I aspirated, I could only eat blended food, and I had to sleep at an angle with lots of pillows. Other than what we were swimming in uncharted waters.

Being right-handed I found it incredibly hard to do simple things like brushing my teeth, washing my face, showering or dressing. Ross had to help me with everything which was a very hard adjustment for me. Being 'Miss Particular', my bedtime routine usually takes half an hour and consists of brushing my teeth, combing the knots out of my hair and counting the grey ones, washing my face and putting on toners, serums and moisturizers which help keep my skin in good condition. I had to quickly learn to do this on my own as I am sure Ross was starting to get a bit fed up by the second week.

I am also very particular when it comes to my living environment in general. The living area and bathrooms must also always be tidy in case an impromptu visitor shows up. Cutlery and crockery must be neatly stored away in the drawers in order of size and shape. Every shelf in the fridge has its purpose, I don't just randomly cram things in there as I like to be able to find things easily. I hated having dirty dishes lying in the sink and always washed them as soon as I was finished cooking. I was therefore frustrated that I couldn't keep everything the way I used to.

I managed to access my private mobile number after a few days and was already inundated with lots of WhatApp texts including a few from clients. I blocked the texts from clients, leaving the office to deal with them, and had the daunting task of explaining to a few close family friends what had happened. I wanted to be able to control the narrative and tell people when I was ready, but there were a few people who were close to me that I felt should know, and I trusted to keep my secret.

I knew I couldn't keep my secret buried forever so I made a list of trusted friends that I should confide in. A childhood friend who I had known for more than 30 years and considered more of a sister than a friend, was one of the first people I told. Our old neighbours had become like an extension of our family over the years, and they too were informed about my stroke.

A very good friend of my sister and I was very shocked when she heard the news. She had only just recovered herself from an illness and we had been planning to meet up to welcome her back home, before my stroke happened. We had a short chat on the phone one week after I was discharged and she made me smile with her office drama stories. She was extremely supportive and called Lulu every day to enquire about my health.

Then there was an old friend from my boarding school days in the UK who I had known since we were 13 years old. I was in Nairobi earlier in the year attending her dear sister's funeral and we promised to stay in touch and meet up again soon. The news of my stroke must have been a massive shock to her, and, though she was still mourning her sister's loss, she checked on me every day and made sure I was always in her prayers. Other close boarding school friends and a very good friend from university also contacted me directly or through Ross offering their support and encouragement.

Another good friend of mine who I first met in law school was also contacted by Ross. I was the older, uncool mature student but my friend had always been kind to me. We kept in contact after law school and she came to stay with me in Tanzania for three months not long after we graduated, and came to Bali for my 40th birthday.

My former kickboxing trainers kept in touch daily and reminded me how strong I was physically and to use that strength in the physiotherapy sessions. Their encouragement made me realise that I was brave enough to face the world, even if it meant being stared at and judged by people.

Everyone I spoke to was shocked, as I was the fittest person they knew. Whilst there are known causes of strokes such as high blood pressure, high cholesterol and diabetes, strokes can happen to anyone. There are cases of young children being affected and more and more people in their 40s are having strokes in Tanzania, partly due to the stress in people's lives, especially women who want to become more financially independent.

Ross was becoming concerned that I was spending too much time on my phone having to explain over and over again what happened. It was difficult at first because each time I answered questions, I kept reliving the event. I knew it had to be done though for me to agreed and come to terms with my new life.

I tried to adjust to my situation but found it incredibly frustrating. Ross cut out the alphabet in small letters and lay them randomly on the dining table. We practised recapping the different letters and he would test my spelling by asking me to spell all the places we had been to together on vacation and the food we ate. Other times I could sit on the sofa watching cooking shows on Netflix, remembering the days when I used to try out new recipes and post them on Instagram. I tried to read books, since I had decided to temporarily switch off both my Facebook and Instagram accounts, but I got distracted very easily. I tried watching my favourite legal drama series but the minute I stopped watching it, reality would sink in and I knew there was no way I would be back practising law any time soon.

Two weeks after returning home it was time for my first outpatient appointment. I went to the hospital with some family members and Ross, and as I sat in the waiting area, I hoped that the doctor would have some answers for me. Why had this happened to me? Why was I getting flashbacks of my stroke? How long would my recovery take? Why was I feeling so sad and angry?

Dr Aris spent fifteen minutes reading through my discharge sheet and all the test results before he spoke to us and conducted a variety of strength and reflex tests.

One thing I remembered vividly from the session was a comment made by a family member to Dr Aris saying to him, "She keeps crying all the time about what hap- pened". I felt very hurt by this comment. How could the person possibly know what I was going through emotionally and mentally?

Thousands of stroke survivors all over the world have cried a lot following their diagnosis, be it tears of disbelief, frustration or otherwise. Instead of chastising me for crying, the family member should have tried to understand my pain. There are many articles online about strokes and stroke recovery. One only needs to do a little research on the subject, and then ask Dr Aris to confirm or clarify what one has read.

My whole world had come to a complete standstill. I had lost all sense of feeling, I had a speech impairment, I lost all mobility on the right side of my body, I had very limited control, and I had lost my ability to earn a living. A similar comment was made a few days later, saying that illness was just something that we can pass through in life, trivialising my condition by comparing it to a knee operation. I too had undergone knee surgery many years ago to fix a torn meniscus. The two conditions are completely different from one another, and recovery from a stroke is far, far more complicated.

I became upset and Ross put a protective hand over me as if to say "don't worry, I am here." Dr Aris was quick to point out that there was no point ruminating over why it happened. I should try to stay positive and focus on my recovery through physiotherapy. Ross asked him if he could it would be a good idea for me to see a psychiatrist and he responded that there was no need. I should just surround myself with close friends or family who will help me get over it. Ross asked a second time thinking maybe Dr Aris had misunderstood him the first time. "No. It is not the African way", he replied. Ross told Lulu about the consultation and lack of support for my state of mind.

When we got home that evening I had my blended food, took my blood thinners and mood enhancer which also doubled as a sedative. The problem with the sedative was that it knocked me out for three hours and then left me awake and anxious for the rest of the night. This had been going on since I had been discharged from hospital. Then one night something worse happened. I was awake at midnight feeling very agitated. My right hand, which had been limp all this time, was at an angle with the muscles all tensed all. Ross came in to check on me and knew something was wrong when I was not able to follow his finger with my eyes.

We ended up at the emergency department once again where the attending doctor kept me under observation for two hours. My blood pressure was elevated and I was extremely cold. Other than that all my vitals were normal and the doctor confirmed that I had had an anxiety attack.

Thinking the mood enhancers were responsible for triggering the attack, I immediately stopped taking them and refused all medication except for the blood thinners.

Ross and Lulu decided it was time to seek professional support for my mental health and began reaching out to their networks to look for a psychiatrist.

CHAPTER FIVE

Rehabilitation

"In rehabilitation there is no elevator. You have to take every step meaning one step at a time."

- Joerg Teichmann

I resumed physiotherapy and speech therapy at home with my therapist PT. Joseph Kisima, a gentle, kind natured and understanding soul. I did not take my sessions seriously in the beginning as I was still in denial about my condition and didn't think much of his involvement in my life at the time. I was in a daze, waiting for the moment when I would wake up from this horrible nightmare.

Many people underestimate the importance of physio- therapy, which plays a key role in the recovery process. Like all treatments, physiotherapy requires time and patience.

Family members should not impose their expectations or timetable on the stroke survivor, rather this needs to be worked out between the physiotherapist and the survivor. They need to discuss and agree on session frequency, desired outcomes and goals, and share the plan with their family.

Unlike a gym membership when you can cancel or skip training sessions, you can not do that with physiotherapy. You cannot simply cancel a session in order to participate in social engagements, it doesn't work like that.

Joseph gave me a great example of the importance of physiotherapy. He said "imagine you had a major surgery and the doctors had prescribed some medication for you to take to help with the recovery. You may choose to in crease or decrease the dose based on the doctor's orders, but you can't say I'm not going to take any medication today because I plan on going out to a bar tonight."

If for whatever reason the physiotherapist is unable to see you, they will provide you with exercises which you can do unsupervised, and with encouragement from family members. My nephew always insisted that I send him videos of the sessions I had with Joseph and would go over them with me when we met.

Being born in the golf capital of the world, St Andrew's in Scotland, Ross knew a thing or two about golfing, and taught my nephew how to use a putter. My nephew in turn helped me work on my right hand gripping skills so we could have friendly putting matches when he came over.

My nephew also played an integral part in improving my speech. When I met with Dr Abeyabo after a few months, I mentioned my speech and asked him if he had any tips to help me regain my accent. He suggested I record myself reading out loud and make sure I correct all the consonants. I tried doing this a few times but didn't like hearing the sound of my voice.

So one day I decided to recruit my nephew to assist me. It was perfect because he was learning to read at school, so we started reading children's books and recording ourselves to make sure every word was pronounced clearly.

I looked forward to my physiotherapy sessions and was disappointed when the floods from the seasonal rains interrupted our time together. At first, Joseph would help me climb the stairs leading up to the other apartments, and I was exhausted after going up and down 160 stairs twice. A few weeks later we were doing six rounds every session covering a total of 480 stairs, doing 70 squats and three sets of bicycle crunches. Soon we got up to 800 steps per session and I felt like Rocky Balboa when he made it to the top of the steps of the Philadelphia Museum of Art.

I pushed myself hard during these sessions, even on the days that I did not feel like it. I could visibly see the improvements each week as the feeling in my limbs and range of motion slowly returned. Not only was I becoming physically stronger, my mental health received a boost too.

CHAPTER SIX

Relationships

"There is only one rule for being a good talker – learnto listen."

- Christopher Morley

Establishing a good relationship with your physiotherapist goes hand in hand with the recovery process. A similar relationship should be established between the family members and carers and the physiotherapist, so they can be updated weekly on the stroke survivor's progress and goals.

A friendship soon developed with Joseph, not only because he was entrusted with my physical recovery, but because I felt I could be completely honest with him about my personal struggles and my recovery in general.

The first lesson I learnt from Joseph was the importance of having a positive attitude towards recovery. He told me a story about two patients of his, one who before the stroke was a healthy man and the other who was overweight. The overweight patient recovered very quickly using lots of positive energy while the healthy one took longer to recover. He had sunk into a depression and couldn't accept what had happened. It was enough motivation for me and I realised I needed to resolve to put in the hard work if I wanted to get better, and decided to put to good use the discipline that I had learned from kickboxing.

What impressed me about Joseph was the passion he had for his craft. He was great at teaching me about how the brain works, how my body had been affected by the injury and how each affected leg, arm and hand muscle had to be retrained then strengthened. It was like I was back in school again and even though I never liked biology, I found his lessons very interesting.

Joseph is at least 10 years younger than me but has a maturity beyond his years. We discussed the upcoming presidential elections in Tanzania and the US, my up- bringing in the UK, my career, his plans for the future, the effect of internet disruption on the general public and why my British accent, which had taken 11 years to perfect, had disappeared overnight.

There were times when I got emotional because of something upsetting that happened and I would break down in tears in the stairwell and lose my balance. He would console me, gently but firmly. "It isn't the right time to bring this up," he would remind me. "Look at how far we have come. We don't need negative energy like that and I don't want you to be thinking negative thoughts after the session."

I learnt a lot from him about the growing need in Tanzania to raise awareness of the condition and he is one of the people who inspired me to tell my story. "Make sure they know that you wrote it all with your left hand!", he advised me.

When it comes to awareness of strokes, many people, especially those from the coastal regions, believe that the condition arises as a result of being hexed, bewitched or cursed. In these regions, when a person has a stroke the first thing the relatives do is to take the patient to a witch doctor or some religious person who specializes in such matters. No brain scans are conducted to identify the cause. Medical treatment is only sought if the witch doctor is unsuccessful. I myself toyed for a brief moment with the idea that something sinister may have been at play, since my mother's family came from the coastal town of Tanga. But common sense and science took over, because I know that if I had entertained any other ideas, they would affect me mentally and hinder my recovery.

People's negative attitude to strokes can also affect the patient's recovery and acceptance of their condition. There is a lot of stigma attached to strokes and many people view it as a disability and would rather keep the stroke survivor locked up at home than encourage them to get out and about. That is why it is essential for stroke survivors to be in a supporting and nurturing environment.

Although Dr Aris had encouraged me to talk to friends, Joseph thought it was too soon at this stage for me to have visitors. Lucy Sondo had also warned me at the hospital about entertaining visitors and that I should focus on rest and recovery. Joseph also suggested I work with my siblings to try and bring back childhood memories which could also help with the recovery process.

I also felt overwhelmed with my family coming to visit at random times which meant I never had any alone time for myself or time to rest during the day. Phone calls were being made in loud voices in my presence and there was nothing I could do as the anger emotion was simply not there. It was all getting out of hand, especially since I was having trouble sleeping, so he recommended that I only see one family member a day a day to give me time to rest during the afternoons.

I conveyed this to my family and a degree of order was temporarily restored with mobile phones being switched off or put on silent mode whenever they visited.

CHAPTER SEVEN

Hope

"You either get bitter or you get better. It's that simple. You either take
what has been dealt to you and allow it to make you a better person, or you
allow it to tear you down. The choice does not belong to fate, it belongs to
you."

– Josh Shipp

With no prospect of going back to work any time soon, I had to think of ways to keep myself busy. I started a gratitude journal, an idea that was inspired by an episode of the Oprah Winfrey show from many years ago when she encouraged people to take up journaling. I didn't take it seriously at the time but now, twelve years later, I remembered her advice.

Every night before going to bed Ross helped me write down a minimum of three things that happened during the day that I was grateful for, and we would stick them on the wall with Post It notes. There were plenty of things I was grateful for which I would have taken for granted in the past. Every few days my father delivered my favourite meal, sweet plantain, which blends very well as baby food. Going for short walks outside the apartment complex or walking around the garden in the evening sunshine. Receiving flowers from an international law firm I worked with for years and well wishes from people that worked with Ross. I even managed a short drive around the Peninsula to survey the damage after three days of heavy rain.

I suggested to my sister one day that we should organise special Muslim prayers ('duas') in the hope that I would take some comfort from the verses of the Qur'an. I remember getting into an argument with Lulu around the dua itself. Every dua is, according to Lulu, incomplete and your prayer will not be received until vast amounts of incense or oud are scattered around. This is a problem for an asthmatic as smoke is one of the key triggers. A compromise was reached in the end where a small amount of oud was scattered. Surely given that I was asthmatic and had suffered a stroke, if Allah is indeed compassionate, he would hear my prayers without the need for excessive use of oud.

During the dua the holy men asked me to say a silent prayer asking God to return me to the condition I was in before the stroke. I prayed for strength to become a better version of my old self, a wiser person who takes better care of herself and puts her needs first ahead of others'.

After the dua, my father sat me down and suggested that I use the recovery period to learn the Qur'an. He explained how learning Arabic and the Qur'an helped him deal with the grief after the death of my mother. He thought it would be a good thing to do 'instead of watching TV all day'.

What he failed to take into account was that firstly I had never been a particularly religious person and I was not about to start now just because something major had happened in my life. I would learn the Qur'an in my own time if I chose to. Secondly, I couldn't learn the Arabic alphabet when I had no movement in my right hand. Thirdly, learning the Qur'an was not an appropriate option at that time as I was struggling with my own demons, and needed plenty of rest. Thankfully Lulu intervened and told him not to force the issue.

It was later that evening I decided I was going to use my time wisely and do something meaningful by writing an account of my experience. I felt it was important for the world to understand what a stroke survivor goes through. I still couldn't remember my laptop password so I started writing on my phone. Ross suggested I use a speech typing software but I knew that that would only frustrate me further since I still couldn't speak properly, so I was adamant about using my left hand to type.

The days were filled with things to do, be it learning to write with my left hand, relearning the alphabet, working on this book or watching our new neighbours (migrating birds) move into the bird boxes that hung out on the balcony.

Lulu came to visit me every day after dropping off AJ at school. AJ got used to my condition although he kept telling his mother that he missed my smile. Some days Lulu would bring along AJ's sweet natured nanny, Mariam Mazengo, who would cook a few days' worth of food at a time and blend it all into what resembled baby food. Lulu and Ross took turns to feed me when she was over during the day and AJ would joke that Mummy is feeding Baby Tee.

Since I was not allowed any water, Ross would make me fresh juices, and smoothies with dates, almond milk, bananas and protein powder. My medication had to be ground to a powder and mixed with a little bit of water, and it often took a couple of minutes to swallow each pill.

My father would visit sometimes during lunchtime, in the evenings after work or before returning home to break his fast. My youngest brother would do the same and my middle brother, who was still in Arusha, called Ross daily to enquire about my progress. The physiotherapy sessions were also going very well and there was movement returning in my right arm.

But when nightfall arrived I would become anxious and not look forward to going to sleep. I was trying to sleep naturally but would lay awake until around 4 am, frustrated. I confided in Ross that my current bedroom was making me very nervous and I was afraid to sleep in case the stroke happened again. We moved to another room but I was still having problems sleeping.

The lack of sleep was unbearable and went on for two weeks. Physical recovery from a stroke depends on a lot of rest which I wasn't getting even during the day. Ross, who was looking after me all this time, was also suffering from exhaustion.

During the earlier weeks, he would wake me up every day, help me into the bathroom and sit me down on a little stool that he bought and bathe me. He would then brush my teeth and patiently go through my beauty routine with me, help me get dressed, brush my hair, sit me down with a glass of fresh juice that he made from scratch and then shower. Ross is a firm believer in meditation and encouraged me to use apps to help me relax. We tried audiobooks, mindfulness and meditation, and they all helped to an extent.

There was one night when I was totally drained from lack of sleep. Overcome with emotion I started crying so hard I was howling like a wounded animal. My throat muscles were still weak and I felt as if my lungs would collapse. I missed my mother so much and yearned for her presence. Boarding school taught me to be independent so I never went to my mother when I was ill, but now I needed her more than ever.

I spoke to my sister the next day about how much I missed our mother. We tried to imagine what it would have been like had she been here and knew we had to learn to cope without her.

My sister and Ross watched me like a hawk, questioning every move I made even when I was simply going to the bathroom. On the day I got my period, my sister hadn't arrived yet at the flat and my right hand was still very weak with no finger movement. I didn't have any choice but to tell Ross what happened. He wasn't embarrassed at all and asked me to explain to him how to put on a sanitary pad. He took me to have a shower and was not in the slightest bit repulsed when blood was pouring down my leg and I kept apologising to him. "There is no need to apologise" he said. "Just show me how to put this on".

PART III

ACCEPTANCE

CHAPTER EIGHT

Mental Battles

"The strongest people are those who win battles weknow nothing about."

– Unknown

A lot of people think that stroke recovery simply involves rehabilitation of the limbs and speech, but this is really just the tip of the iceberg. As the brain reboots it is very common to experience a change in emotions and behaviour. As stroke survivors' bodies readjust they may experience fits of rage, anger or try to blame themselves or others for their condition. Carers and family members should be aware that this change in behaviour is to be expected and bear in mind that it is an integral part of the recovery process, taking place alongside the physical rehabilitation.

Ross spent a lot of time reading articles about what to expect during the stroke recovery process and was aware that there would likely be some behavioural changes. Instead of screaming and shouting out of frustration, I could cry a lot or just internalise my emotions, which was worse. I can compare my experience to that of a new born baby. At first the baby cries all the time, often for no reason at all. When it gets to the terrible twos, the baby starts throwing tantrums because of frustration and because the parent isn't listening to it. As the child gets older it learns to control its emotions and develops a personality. So, imagine you're going through all this and at the same time learning to walk, speak, swallow and do all the very basic skills that you once learned as a child. This is stroke recovery.

Ross accepted all these changes without complaining and learned to accommodate my needs and wishes. I was a stroke patient after all and needed a calm and nurturing environment without any negativity that could hinder my progress.

I was making good progress physically and started to get some movement in my right arm, but still couldn't sleep at night. Ross read articles about post stroke anxiety and found something linking strokes to posttraumatic stress disorder (PTSD), particularly when the patient is fully conscious during the stroke episode, as I had been. He immediately got in touch with a friend of his who was an army Major during the Afghanistan war and had suffered from severe PTSD. His friend explained that he had managed to get rid of 80% of the PTSD through a form of psychotherapy known as EMDR (Eye Movement Desensitization and Reprocessing) that enables people to heal from the symptoms and emotional distress that are the result of traumatic incidents. He and Lulu got in touch with a friend who put them in contact with a counsellor and a psychiatrist.

Ross had an initial telephone consultation with Dr Praexida Swai and explained my situation. The top priority was for me to get some rest, as I was suffering from exhaustion due to lack of sleep caused by the nightly anxiety. I had always liked to be in control of my body and never liked filling it with lots of medication I wouldn't even take a painkiller unless it was absolutely necessary. It was important that whatever medication Dr

Praexida prescribed would not leave me feeling drowsy all day and knock me out at night.

I was very nervous when we arrived at Dr Praexida's office. She had already informed Ross prior to our meeting that she practised EMDR and I didn't know what to expect from the sessions. Dr Praexida has a very gentle and calming voice. I automatically relaxed as soon as she started speaking.

She explained that having panic attacks after a stroke was very common and quickly confirmed that I was suffering from PTSD. She pointed out the importance of having plenty of sleep as it played a significant part in the recovery process.

Dr Praexida went on to discuss the medication that she would prescribe, which were mood enhancers that would also improve energy levels and reduce my anxiety, which in turn would also help with sleeping. I tensed up as soon as she mentioned sleeping pills as I was afraid of a repeat of what happened with the previous medication. I tried to make light of the situation and said "Can you give me something that gently lulls me to sleep, like when you have a glass of white wine. Not something that knocks me out cold the entire night. I want to be able to wake up if I need to use the bathroom, or in case there is a fire." She smiled understandably and suggested I take a quarter of the tablet which was 0.5 mg. "But you need to have a positive attitude to the medication" she warned me, "in order for them to take effect. Don't try to reject them from your body"

Nighttime came and even though I had finished getting ready for bed I kept trying to postpone the inevitable. I slowly got into bed and Ross gave me the mood enhancer first, which was supposed to take effect after 4 weeks. As soon as I took the antianxiety tablet, I would feel it travelling through the body. I got up in a panic and Ross dragged me back into bed. "Don't try to fight it, just stay calm. Don't worry I am here." "Please stay with me until I fall asleep" I pleaded with him. "I'm not going anywhere," he assured me.

He started reminiscing about our trip to Italy last year and all the delicious food we had eaten. I also reminded him of some of the places we visited and how happy I was on that trip. I soon started yawning and gently fell asleep.

Nine hours later I woke up feeling extremely rested. "How did you sleep", Ross asked. "Very well," I replied with a smile.

After three good nights of decent sleep I started to see more changes in my body. I felt brighter, was able to drink a smoothie from a glass and not a cup like a baby and even managed to give Ross a one and a half-armed hug. Progress at last!

Ross would recall the day's events to me when I was trying to fall asleep and started reading to me through gritted teeth one of the chick literature books. He is a bit of a literary snob and soon convinced me to switch to a classic Around the World in 80 Days, which I enjoyed.

The following week, having had the initial consultation, I was very nervous about my first EMDR session and I had no idea what to expect. Would Dr Praexida hypnotize me and uncover hidden characteristics from centuries ago? She assured me that there was no hypnosis involved and asked me to think of a memory from a place that I had visited in the past which made me feel safe.

EMDR turned out to be a kind of rapid physiotherapy for the mind, and I was able to desensitize my traumatic memories of the stroke after just two sessions. I was finally able to walk into my normal bedroom at 3 am to use the bathroom without being scared. Those who are interested on how

EMDR works can find detailed information of the practice here: www.emdr.com/what-is-emdr/

I still had a lot of unresolved issues from my past that had been buried deep inside that I wanted to discuss with Dr Praexida, such as my eating disorder which started at the age of ten, a choking incident involving an exboyfriend that continued to haunt me 23 years later, and the constant search for validation from my father which led to me becoming the perfectionist I no longer wished to be. I continued to see Dr Praexida once a week.

Psychiatry has always been frowned upon in Tanzania and psychiatrists are known as 'head doctors', or doctors that specialise in treating crazy people. It is no wonder people hesitate to see them. What people forget though is that mental wellbeing is equally important, if not more so, than physical fitness. Sometimes you need to discuss matters with a trained professional to help organise your thoughts without judgement.

Family and close friends are not equipped to assist a stroke survivor with the mental battles that they are faced with. That is why seeing a psychiatrist or a counsellor after suffering a major life changing event such as a stroke is so important and a vital aspect of the recovery process.

CHAPTER NINE

Shame

"We live in an atmosphere of shame. We are ashamed of everything that is real about us; ashamed of our- selves, of our relatives, of our incomes, of our ac- cents, of our opinion, of our experience, just as we are ashamed of our naked skins."

- George Bernard Shaw

One of the reasons why I didn't want any visitors in the early days of my recovery was because of shame. My shame was more superficial because we live in a world where appearances are everything. I had been trained from my boarding school days in the UK to be mindful of my general appearance. Accordingly I always made sure I was presentable. I was like a luxury car. The exterior was always polished and shiny, but under the bonnet the engine was beginning to rust and a few parts needed replacing. I didn't want people to see my broken parts.

Having a disability or any kind is still considered taboo in the African community. I had been taught in boarding school to be respectful to people who are physically or mentally impaired, and we were encouraged to socialize and work with disability groups. Every girl was required during the sixth form to spend a week in a care home, as part of a community service program.

I had a feeling that stroke survivors would face a similar challenge of being ostracised from the community in Tanzania. I tried to ask this question in one of the consultations but I didn't get a straight answer. I therefore turned to Joseph since he was already working with more than seven stroke survivors.

Joseph confirmed my suspicions that many stroke survivors were indeed kept indoors pretty much all the time, until they had fully recovered. Some stroke survivors are ashamed because, before the stroke, they had managed to reach a certain level of financial success and wanted their friends to continue to see the positive aspects of their achievements. They are then concerned how their family and community members will view them following the stroke.

Given the fact that a stroke involves damage to brain cells, family members and loved ones may suspect that the stroke survivor will become mentally impaired, especially during the early stages of recovery when the survivor cannot speak or respond to questions. A further reason why a family member or loved ones may feel ashamed is due to their own personal traits. If they are successful members of their community and have reputations to uphold, they may think that if they admit that there is a problem in their family, other members of the community will believe that the person needs some sort of financial assistance. Therefore the family member or loved one would rather handle the problem on their own, rather than confide in others who in actual fact may be able to provide some much needed emotional support.

Unfortunately I suffer from cabin fever, especially when I am sick, so after a week of being stuck indoors I ventured out into the compound garden and bumped into neighbours. They were all very sympathetic and wanted to help in whatever way they could.

I felt encouraged and one day I asked Ross to take me outside onto our street which is usually pretty quiet. It was boiling hot and I felt uncomfortable in the wheel chair, but I didn't care. I was out in the open watching cars driving by.

Most days Ross would go to the shops only if Lulu was around to watch me. I convinced him to take me with him one day and told him I would just stay in the car while he was in the supermarket. The next day when my family heard about my little excursion, I could sense that they were not pleased.

Support from family members and loved ones when it comes to handling shame is so important. Being ashamed of their condition and keeping stroke survivors locked indoors does not help them with their recovery in any way. The family should be grateful for the fact that the person survived the stroke, and encourage the survivor to go out into the world and be surrounded by nature or the ocean.

I was reminded of a story that my mother told me many years ago. She was a committee member for the Tanzania Paralympics Team and would often travel to parts of the country to scout for potential members for the Team. She was once in a small town and heard rumours of a woman who had locked up her child.

My mother went to a house with a member of the local authority and discovered a physically impaired child who had been kept indoors for years. They took the child outside and he rubbed his eyes trying to adjust to the daylight.

The Paralympics coaches took him to the local athletics field and discovered that he was very good at running. They continued to train the child and several months later he returned to his mother's house in a suit, having represented Tanzania at the Paralympics. The mother was delighted for her son's new found freedom, talent and success.

On the day of my 43rd birthday, Ross suggested that we go for sundowners at a nearby hotel that overlooked the Indian Ocean. I reluctantly agreed, put on a nice blue dress and tried my best to look normal.

The moment we entered the restaurant I felt a million eyes on me. Everyone was staring at me as Ross guided me to our table. For a second I felt ashamed and wanted to leave. But my inner voice told me "You're not leaving. You have worked so hard to get this far, and no one has the right to take that away from you, or judge you." So, I held my head high and slowly walked to our table. I spoke to the waiter who was attending to us, Gaudence. He was very kind, helping me choose a smoothie that I could drink, and said he would pray for me at mass that Sunday.

Undeterred by that experience, a few days later, I decided to go to a nearby shopping centre. I had been going there for years and almost all the shop owners knew my name. At first, they didn't recognise me as I had a mask on and was wearing glasses instead of my usual contact lenses. I had also lost a lot of weight. They were all very sympathetic when they heard my story, telling me I will get better very soon and that they would pray for me. I never knew it was possible to feel so much love from people I didn't know all that well. I left the shopping centre with a full heart, encouraged by the well wishes and felt alive again. From that day onwards I went shopping with Ross or Lulu, walking into shops like a normal person instead of hiding with shame.

Once I got over the shame it motivated me to work harder on my recovery. It took me a while to really accept my condition, and in one of the sessions with Joseph I confessed that I felt much happier now because I had become comfortable with my current state.

I am not embarrassed about my body and I don't see myself as a disabled person. Now whenever I get up I notice I walk faster, straighter and not hunched over as much on my right side, and look back with pride at all the progress I have made.

CHAPTER TEN

Empathy

"Empathy is simply listening, holding space, withholding judgment, emotionally connecting, and communicating that incredibly healing message of you're not alone."

- Brene Brown

One of my brothers was still in Arusha following my stroke, and attended to some business in Nairobi before flying down to Dar to see me. He did ask Ross to keep him abreast daily of any developments, and was careful to self isolate for a few days before visiting me. He was mindful of the need to respect my rest periods and physiotherapy sessions and therefore arranged to visit at a time that was convenient for me.

Ross showed him pictures of my hospital stay and explained to him what I had gone through. I told him that I was certain that stress played a role in contributing to the stroke, and that he too should try and take better care of his health.

Being a business minded person, he asked me if I had considered finding someone to manage my law firm, and whether I still enjoyed being a lawyer. He also suggested when I was better I should spend some time at a wellness retreat, to help me get away from Tanzania and to recharge.

He was aware through the chats that we had in the family WhatsApp group that I had been sick for a while. When he came to see me he apologised and said that the family should have taken me more seriously, as the warning signs were there.

Even though my voice was tired from all that talking, I allowed my brother to stay awhile, as I could see that he was genuinely interested in knowing more about my condition and well being.

He went on to introduce me to another stroke survivor, Sofia-Magdalena Karlsson. Sofia had an ischaemic stroke when she was 26 years old. She had had no preexisting conditions and, like me, the cause of the stroke remains unknown. The first sign of the stroke she had was the loss of her eyesight. She lost all sight on the left side of both eyes, resulting in the loss of 75% of her field of vision. She also lost the ability to see depth and space, and her ability to notice the passing of time.

She went to the hospital immediately when the stroke happened, but was sent home as the doctors thought she just had a migraine. She went back and forth to the hospital over a period of four days and was sent home on each occasion.

The doctors finally agreed to do a CT scan and found that she had indeed had a stroke. She was admitted to the hospital as an inpatient, only to be discharged the day after due to a terrorist attack in Oslo, as she had to make way for those injured by the attack.

Sofia was bedridden for the next 8 months, and she did not receive enough support from her then husband and in-laws. Sofia was expected to be "normal" but there was nothing normal about the situation she was in. She suffered from panic attacks due to severe PTSD, and had no one around her that was even close to understanding what she was going through.

Sofia's story stuck with me for days, and despite being incredibly saddened by her experience, I was inspired by her bravery. She still had faith in the human race despite what had happened to her. She reminded me that there is so much love out there, even if we are let down by those closest to us.

Around mid-November Ross brought up the subject of going back to Scotland. He had been in Tanzania since August and his extended visa was about to expire. He also wanted to check on his parents in Edinburgh. I knew that he was exhausted and in need of some time off to rest and process the events of the past two months.

I wrote to his parents updating them of my progress and let them know that Ross would be back soon. I didn't anticipate that it would be in two weeks, so when he broke the news to me, I naturally broke down in tears. A family member mistook the sobbing for a breakdown on my part that needed to be resolved quickly, meaning I needed to toughen up.

Ross and I had been through so much over the past two months that it was natural for me to become emotionally attached to him when I saw that he was the only one who genuinely comforted and consoled me during my lows.

I discussed the situation with Dr Praexida and she offered some very useful tips which immediately lifted my spirits and helped me realise that I would be able to cope during his absence. I was eager to share these tips with my family after the session but instead of listening and being supportive, family members said I was becoming too emotionally attached to Ross. The tough love attitude that they exhibited was the opposite of the emotional support I needed from them.

I tried to distract myself online and to process how their comments made me feel That is when I stumbled across a Harvard Business Review article by Vasundhara Sawhey titled 'It's Okay to Not Be Okay' which focuses on toxic positivity. Dr Jaime Zuckerman, a licenced clinical psychologist who Vasundhara interviewed, describes the concept as the assumption that despite a person's emotional pain or difficult situation, they should only have a positive mindset. Dr Zuckermam believes that if a person is not in a positive mood, and we invalidate the person's emotional state, we end up eliciting secondary emotions inside them like shame, guilt and embarrassment.

She explains that "efforts to avoid, ignore or suppress emotions that are appropriate to context can isolate someone in their time of need, thereby perpetuating the stigma that mental health issues equate to weakmindedness".

Dr Zuckerman suggests that instead of using phrases like "positive vibes only" or "what's there to cry about. It'll be fine", people should use phrases that affirm the other person's emotions and let them know you are here to support them without expectation. "Not only is it okay not to feel 'okay'" she says "it is essential. An abnormal emotional response to an abnormal situation IS normal. We cannot simply pick the emotions we want to have".

I reached out to an old friend, Fanny Nyembwe, who had had breast cancer three years previously and understood all too well about the pain and suffering that comes with battling an illness, and the need to be surrounded by empathetic people. Her sage advice had kept me going through the days when I was very emotional and felt misunderstood. She confirmed that it was okay to own your feelings and be upset when your world has been turned upside down.

CHAPTER ELEVEN

Compassion

"Empathy is the capacity to "share" the feelings of others while compassion is the capacity to not only share feelings but also feel compelled to alleviate their suffering. The difference between empathy and compassion shows up in emotional reactions, especially when faced with someone in pain".

- Hiroyuki Miyazaki

I was fortunate enough during my recovery to have all my medication and financial needs taken care of by my father and sister. However, looking after a patient, no matter what their condition, requires more than being there for them financially. The family can't simply hire a team of professionals to fix you without playing an active role themselves in the recovery process or to try and understand the challenges that the stroke survivor is likely to encounter along the way.

The patient needs an environment where they can trust you with their feelings and thoughts, and you need to be aware of their constant change of moods, and their need for emotional support. This was why I was able to get along very well with Ross and my cousin Asha, because they were able to read my mind and know instantly what was bothering me and how to make me feel better.

This is one of the biggest challenges that stroke survivors face during the recovery the lack of compassion from their family members and friends. I spoke to several stroke survivors and heard stories of family members who were too harsh with them, berated them or offered little or no support. Common reasons for this can be put down to a failure to fully understand the condition, denial or simply an unwillingness to accept that their loved one has changed, and, of course, shame.

I have had to deal with challenging family dynamics instead of focusing on my recovery. In the beginning, I tried to send some reading material about the challenges of stroke recovery to my family, hoping it would give them some guidance on how to support me, but I am not sure if that was sufficient. I highly recommend that family members read the article "13 Things Every Stroke Survivor Wished You Knew", which can be found on the Flint Rehab website, for a better insight of what we go through and how we feel.

Looking after a stroke survivor is not a competition amongst family members. My mother chose my cousin Asha to spend her last months with her over her sisters, for the same reason that I chose Ross to look after me - compassion.

Family members need to respect the survivor's choice of carer, and the rules that the carer sets in place. Requesting family members to respect visiting hours, asking them to knock instead of using the doorbell and requiring them to switch off their phones when they enter the home are rules that are very easy to follow and stick to.

When a physiotherapist works with a stroke survivor they try to help the survivor to get back to doing the things they enjoyed before the stroke, especially if the survivor was into fitness and sports.

Kickboxing was a major part of my life. Not only was it a great stress reliever, but after I was choked by an ex- boyfriend when I was younger, I vowed to learn a form of martial arts that would ensure that I would never allow myself to be hurt again by a man. My physiotherapist knew how much I missed the sport and surprised me in one of our sessions. He got me to put on my boxing gloves and we did some very light punching to help strengthen my right arm. I felt elated after the session, I was so happy and told him that it felt like an early Christmas present.

When I lost the use of my right hand I felt helpless as this was my dominant side. I knew it would be a while before I could use my right hand again so he encouraged me to use my left hand as much as possible. When family members heard this suggestion they were not pleased because culturally the left hand is considered unclean, because it is used for ablutions. Furthermore, according to Islam, only the devil eats with his left hand, so one must never use the left hand for eating, drinking, writing or accepting anything. If Allah was as compassionate and understanding as he is meant to be, surely he would allow me to use whatever means necessary to assist with my recovery.

Despite this cultural norm, I persisted as I was getting tired of being spoon fed all the time. Being able to use my left hand and using it for daily tasks gave me a sense of independence, allowing me to learn to bathe and dress myself, to write, use colouring books for relaxation and even write this book. Family members should encourage stroke survivors to use their

73

working hands as much as possible and even provide tools to assist them with their writing. Once the survivor has regained full use of their dominant hand, they will have gained a useful new skill ambidexterity.

Early in my recovery Ross had to keep a close eye on me and offered me his hand whenever we went out, whether it was to the hospital for a checkup or to the shops. Family members often forget that your movements will be slow and must therefore be patient with you, and try not to rush you. I know chivalry is pretty much dead these days but you have to be aware of it when dealing with a stroke survivor and be aware of any heavy doors that might close on them.

One of the effects of the stroke I continued to experience was fatigue (and still do at the time of writing). A 20 minute trip to the shops or simple activities left me as exhausted as if I had run a marathon, sometimes requiring naps of up to 2 hours to recover. Talking for more than a couple of hours also has the same effect, sapping my energy levels and leaving me drained for the next 24 hours. Many stroke survivors experience this so need more sleep and plenty of rest to allow the brain to regenerate and rewire itself. It is important for family members to take this into account especially after a stroke survivor had spent over two hours at the hospital waiting for a consultation. Any extra trips or tasks on the same day should be avoided.

I was still writing my account on my mobile phone, which was becoming rather tedious and was causing problems with my eyesight. I was still locked out of my laptop and couldn't even sign in as a guest. One of my brothers is a whizz with computers so I asked for his assistance. He managed to partition the hard drive and create a new profile for me, allowing me to continue writing but now with the familiarity of a proper keyboard.

One day my nephew came to visit and I was lying on the sofa relaxing. All of a sudden he grabbed a paper napkin. He disappeared off into one of the bathrooms and reappeared, having applied some water to it. Without any prompting from me, he started wiping my right hand and leg very gently. I asked him what he was doing and he said he was trying to make me better.

Another incident I will never forget was when one of my brothers spent the night at my apartment. Ross told me that two of his friends were in town for a short visit. He hadn't had a day off from looking after me since the stroke happened and wanted to meet up with them to watch rugby Scotland were playing. He asked one of my brothers if he would stay the night and watch over me and give me my nightly medications. I wasn't thrilled with the idea when I found out, but knew he needed a break. "It's for one night", I kept telling myself, "and if you feel scared or overwhelmed, just go to your safe place like Dr Praexida taught you."

My brother arrived around 6.30 pm and Ross showed him the medication I take every night and the food I was having that evening. As soon as Ross left, I felt the back of my neck tensing up. This always happened even before the stroke when I was either very stressed or nervous. I started thinking about my safe place, but then stopped myself. Wait a second, I thought to myself this is my kid brother who I had been looking out for since he was a baby. There is nothing scary about him. My sister and I nicknamed him the Gentle Giant as he has a deep voice and a calming presence. He was never on his phone when he came to visit me, always listened, never interrupted and asked thoughtful questions at the right moments.

The only way to stay calm and not freak out was to talk to him, which I did. We talked about work, marriage, and how he shouldn't feel pressured to do so until he was absolutely ready. We also talked about our mother, and how he was coping following my stroke.

When it was time for dinner he warmed up my blended food and patiently fed me until I had had enough. Al- though I kept it to myself I was overcome with emotion, seeing how gentle he was with me. I had flashbacks of when he was a baby and how I, being 10 years his senior, used to feed him, but now it was the other way around.

We chatted some more after dinner, discussing lighter topics such as entertainment, with comedy clips from the Trevor Noah show playing in the background. I got ready for bed, using the new electric toothbrush that Ross' friend had brought from Scotland for me. It made brushing my teeth so much easier, and thankfully I didn't have to ask my brother to do this task for me. He patiently waited as I went through the routine of taking 5 minutes to swallow each pill, and stayed by my bedside until the yawns became more frequent, signalling that I would fall asleep soon.

I woke up in the middle of the night in a slight panic as I noticed the bed next to mine was empty. I didn't have my glasses on, but on my way to the bathroom I could make out a figure in the living room and assumed it was my brother watching a movie. I woke a second time at around 6 am and saw him cocooned in a bed sheet and went back to sleep.

By the time I woke up around 9.30 am my brother was already up waiting for me and stayed with us for an extra hour and a half, even though I knew he hadn't slept for long the night before. Later on I thanked Ross for asking my brother to stay overnight as it gave us a chance to really bond and connect.

My former colleague Bart Wilms, who was in town from Dubai also paid me a surprise visit. He was about to start working for a new company and being between jobs had decided to come to Dar es Salaam for a short visit.

He contacted Ross the night before to check if it was okay to call on me.

I have been disappointed many times in the past by people I thought were friends, so I kept my list of friends very short. Bart's presence on the day he was due to fly home lifted my spirits, and reinforced the fact that there are people in the world who do care for others, and I am very blessed to have him as a friend.

PART IV

BRUISED, NOT BROKEN

CHAPTER TWELVE

RegainingControl

"No one has power over you unless you give it to them, you are in control of your life and your choicesdecide your own fate."

- Anonymous

J oseph encouraged me early on in my recovery to speak to other stroke survivors, as their experiences would help me make sense of my own situation, combat my frustrations and give me hope.

I was struggling for weeks to deal with my family as I felt that some of them did not understand what I was going through, or were not being supportive or empathetic about the emotions I was experiencing. I kept being asked every day whether my right hand was working, even though Joseph had previously explained to family members that the hand takes the longest time to heal. I felt like I was being pressured into going back to work too soon, and that they were interfering with my healing process. I reached out for advice to the person who knew me very well, Lucy Sondo.

Although I never lashed out in anger like some stroke survivors, I kept my anger and frustration bottled up inside me, which was worse. Lucy taught me that healing has to start with me, because no one else could possibly know what I am going through. She advised me that I had to let people know gently if they were doing things that were upsetting me instead of bottling everything up. I had to learn to control my emotions, try to get as much rest as possible and find ways to relax. She warned that all of this would not be easy, but that things would settle down in time.

The chat with Lucy really helped me figure out how to regain control of my life and get back to my normal self. I wanted to become an even better version of my former self. That same evening I sent a text to my sister and asked her to arrange a chat with her, my father and I on Friday before he went to the mosque for prayers. I couldn't sleep the night before as I kept going through what I wanted to say to them in my head. I needed them to accept my condition, be more emotionally supportive and most importantly of all, I wanted them to listen to me.

Sensing something serious was about to go down, my father preempted the meeting by turning up at my apart ment on the Thursday evening. I decided to change my strategy a bit because I wanted both of them to be there when I did the discussion. So I started talking to my father about my work, how I had pushed myself so hard over the past 18 years and how exhausting it had been.

I was almost in tears when I explained all this to him. All he saw was a machine that had been running seamlessly for years when in actual fact the engine was shot and I had been running on empty.

The next day I had the meeting with Lulu and my father. Before we began I insisted that they turn off their phones and not interrupt me until I had finished speaking. I told them that I needed them to be more supportive, not financially, but emotionally. I needed them to be more empathetic, listen and try to understand why I was acting a certain way, instead of making their own assumptions and expecting me to align with their expectations.

They had their own views and comments about what I had to say but I did not let them upset me. What was important was that I had finally managed to get a lot off my chest unresolved issues from the past and new ones connected to my stroke. That evening it felt like a huge load had been lifted from my shoulders and I slept peacefully.

CHAPTER THIRTEEN

Learning To Cope

"They always say time changes things, but you actually have to change them yourself"

- Andy Warhol

With two weeks to go before Ross' trip back home, I knew I had to step up and start becoming more independent. It was agreed that my cousin Asha from Zanzibar would come and stay with me while Ross was away.

We had a new hanging shower installed in the bathroom, I dug out my Michael Jackson style shower mitts and Ross supervised me to make sure I showered properly. My right arm would only go up at a 45-degree angle and sometimes hurt when I tried to put on a tee shirt, but I was determined to wash myself. Putting on a bra was an absolute nightmare since the fingers had not learned how to grip small things, use zips or buttons, or lace up my shoes. I persevered.

I started to use my right hand more in my daily activities even though I was starting to become a pro with my left hand. I even surprised Ross once by getting up early and doing the dishes, all with my left hand. As my grip became stronger I started carrying small 500ml water bottles for a short distance. My confidence went overboard one day when I tried to carry an empty glass of water. I barely made it to the kitchen counter when the glass slipped from my hand and fell to the ground, where it shattered into pieces. I froze on the spot, like a child waiting to be scolded by their parent, as I recalled that the blood thinning medication made my blood flow a lot more if I cut myself.

The day of Ross' departure was very difficult for me. We had the whole day together and I wanted us to be left alone. Around 4 pm, some family members came over to spend the night with my cousin Asha and I so we would not feel lonely.

Then, an hour later, more family members arrived. It was all so overwhelming that I went to my bedroom and started crying. Ross calmed me down and we sat alone uninterrupted for half an hour. Later on my nephew wanted to go into the pool so Ross went in with him and they spent an hour together.

As the time to go to the airport approached I tried to hold it together, helping him get ready, wishing I was going with him. As we waited for the Uber to arrive Ross took my nephew to one side and asked him to give me lots of hugs when he left. I managed to contain my emotions as we said goodbye to each other, but as soon as I walked back into the flat I started crying uncontrollably, not caring who saw me. When I went to the bathroom to pull myself together, my nephew followed me, not leaving my side. I apologised to him for crying, and he said "even I had tears in my eyes when Uncle Ross was leaving".

CHAPTER FOURTEEN

Close Companion

"When we honestly ask ourselves which person in our lives means the most to us, we often find that it is those who, instead of giving advice, solutions, or cures, have chosen rather to share our pain and touch our wounds with a warm and tender hand."

— *Henri Nouwen*

My cousin Asha Mtindo is a very strong willed and vivacious person who gets along with everyone.She lures you with her sing-song Zanzibari accent and Comorian roots, which give her a unique beauty. The fact that we both like looking after our skin made us perfect housemates.

Asha was very close to my mother and it was her that my mother chose to look after her when she was sick, even though she had two sisters. Asha also spent two months in Nairobi helping my sister get ready to deliver her first born. Caring for people came naturally to her.

I was a bit apprehensive about her visit, but the minute she walked through the front door I knew everything would be okay. She gave me a massive hug and stood back admiring my progress, saying 'mashallah mashallah' over and over.

Asha is also an incredible cook. For the next two days the apartment was filled with the sweet aroma of Zanzibar spices. She slowly introduced me back to normal food and Ross was treated to very flavoursome meals. She and Ross tried to communicate in broken English and I encouraged him to finally learn Kiswahili so he wouldn't feel left out in our conversations.

I thought my world would fall apart after Ross left, but Asha kept me entertained with tales of the Spice Island. She quickly became more of a companion than a carer to me. She had a rebellious streak which I loved and we laughed so much recalling our childhood days. When we weren't doing charcoal detox facials or watching Christmas movies on TV, we sat outside by the pool shooting the breeze.

She told me she could swim but at first I didn't believe her. Then one day I forced her to put on her swimsuit and prove me wrong. She was a bit nervous at first even though she went swimming early every morning so people wouldn't see her. I assured her that people in the compound kept to themselves, and that nobody would be watching her. Her ability to swim so gracefully left me floored and jealous that I couldn't join her in the pool in my current state.

Some days she would tell me about the time she spent looking after my mother. That gave me some closure because I still had some unresolved issues surrounding her passing that I had been carrying around for 7 years.

I learnt so much from Asha in the three weeks that we spent together. Even though she faced so many adversities in her life, starting with a brief marriage at the age of 15, she still managed to have a positive outlook on life.

I got to learn the cultural heritage of both our families which extended all the way to the Comoros Island and Turkey, making me yearn to visit these places one day. Spending time with Asha made me realise how fortunate my mother and I were to have someone like her looking after us. She must have required so much patience and compassion to care for us both and she did all that as if we were her own blood. I am eternally grateful for hav ing her in my life and look forward to celebrating her 50th birthday with her, inshallah, which coincidentally is the day before the anniversary of my mother's death.

CHAPTER FIFTEEN

Positive Language

"Words have energy and power with the ability to help, to heal, to hinder, to hurt, to harm, to humiliate, and to humble."

— *Yehuda Berg*

The use of positive and encouraging language is very important when dealing with stroke survivors.

Family members and loved ones are strongly encouraged to refrain from commenting on the stroke survivor's appearance during the early stages of recovery, as this is the period where the survivor is in a very vulnerable state. My nephew AJ saw very clearly that there was a physical change in me but he never commented out loud. He would instead tell his mother in private how much he missed my smile.

A family member on the other hand was quick to point out to me one day that my mouth was still deviated to one side. I spent that afternoon examining myself in the bathroom, wondering if there were any other disfigure- ments that I should be aware of. When I told Joseph the next day what happened he sighed and said there is nothing wrong with my mouth.

One should also refrain from making any negative assumptions or remarks about the stroke survivor's carer, especially if the carer is the survivor's life partner. A stroke survivor is already under a lot of pressure following the stroke. How will they earn a living? Will their business cope without their presence? What about their family? Will their spouse stick with them 'in sickness and in health'.

I had no concerns whatsoever that Ross would abandon me in my hour of need. He had already proved to me that he wasn't going anywhere. But a comment made by a family member suggesting that he might leave me was just cruel and unnecessary.

My nephew kept telling me that I would get better in 2 weeks time (bless him). He even said to me in November that I had to get better now. "Why", I asked. "Because it is going to be your birthday soon, like mama". "But I won't be able to have cake as I am still eating baby food", I told him, knowing that this would be my first birthday without cake. "Of course you will," he assured me. "What kind of cake should I get?" "Chocolate" he replied without any hesitation.

On another occasion I was chatting with Asha and found out that she was turning 50 in February 2021. I love a good party, especially when it involves someone reaching a milestone age, so I immediately got excited. I wanted to organise a party in her honour to thank her for all her support and help in caring for my mother and me. Asha encouraged the idea and played along even though she didn't really need any party to celebrate her birthday. What she was doing was using positive language to encourage me and offer me some hope so that one day I would be fit enough to do anything I wanted, including hosting a party.

One day I had a chat with my nephew and tried to explain to him what happened to me. I told him that I was working very hard to get better so that we could spend time together again like we used to. I promised that I would do my best but told him that I would need his help to get better.

It upset me not spending time and playing with my nephew. Each time Ross reminded me that this would happen again soon.

Joseph told me a story of a female stroke survivor whose own mother had passed away from a stroke. She was convinced that the same would happen to her. Her family did not help matters as they too thought that she would succumb to the condition. She therefore did not see any point in making an effort with her physiotherapy sessions. What was the point as she fully expected to die? Unfortunately the stroke survivor died in the end from asphyxiation which occurred during her recovery. Perhaps her premature passing could have been avoided had the family provided support and positivity.

CHAPTER SIXTEEN

Peace and Tranquility

"A few moments of inner peace and quiet allows the brain to reset itself.
You become more centered as this happens, since the brain is clearing out
distractions and too much 'cross talk'"

- Deepak Chopra

When someone asks me if I am feeling better or wishes me a speedy recovery, I sometimes find such statements difficult to respond to, because it's not like I am recovering from a cold. There is no such thing as a speedy recovery for stroke survivors, and friends and loved ones need to be aware of this.

Before Ross left for the UK he asked me to talk to Asha to make sure that my family respected the boundaries that he had tried to instill. This was to ensure that I got as much rest as possible.

Asha was able to stick to the plan the first couple of days and then things began to deteriorate. Family members arranged for repair men to come into the flat to fix this and that and on one occasion, without any prior notice, carpenters showed up to remove and re varnish my front door.

I refused to leave as there was no way I was going to leave my apartment unguarded without a door. In all the commotion of trying to figure out how I wanted my door varnished, I went up the stairs to look at one of my neighbour's doors but missed a step and fell onto the stair. Luckily I fell on my left side and caught the railing with my left hand, so only bruised the bottom of my chin and not my head.

There was also the issue of eating. Even before my stroke I never found enough quiet time to sit down and enjoy my lunch. People always chose lunchtime to call or come over to see me for work, so I ended up eating a few forkfuls at a time and throwing away the rest since my appetite had been ruined. The fact that I had an eating disorder, which gets worse whenever something major happens in my life did not help either. I lost weight when my paternal grandmother passed away, and again when my mother passed away.

Forcing food down my throat every couple of hours like a Thanksgiving turkey, and weighing me every week, only stressed me out more. It was normal after all for any patient to lose some weight when they are in hospital, and it takes time for them to get back to normal.

In order to try and create a relaxing environment which would allow me to eat in peace, Ross and I created a 'no speaking at the dinner table' rule. This rule was crucial as it also allowed me to focus on chewing my food properly when I was back to eating solid food there by reducing the risk of choking.

Asha tried to enforce this rule and would leave me to eat in peace either in the dining room, or in her room if there were visitors over. Some family members didn't like this rule and insisted one day that I eat at the dining table with them.

What they failed to realise was that I found any background noise such as phone calls very off putting and would end up losing my appetite and throwing my food in the bin when no one was looking. I needed all the calories I could get, primarily so that my brain could use the energy to repair the body.

When I did manage to have a peaceful and quiet day where I could have more rest, it filled me with energy and meant that I could be much better equipped for physiotherapy sessions as well as carrying out other hobbies and tasks assigned by Joseph.

CHAPTER SEVENTEEN

Holidays

"The people in your life should be a source of reducing stress, not causing more of it."

- The Good Vibe

Ross had hoped that I would end my book on a positive note with the family all gathered at Christmas but I had the feeling that things would not go as smoothly as he imagined.

The holidays are a stressful time for everyone. There is pressure on families to come together and catch up on their achievements for the year. Traditionally most Tanzanian families celebrate Christmas in their homes and often invite neighbours and other relatives over. This is what we used to do growing up.

As the years went by and an upper middle class emerged, the traditional ways were replaced with lavish parties and Christmas lunches at 5 star hotels. Families mingled in their fancy clothes, displaying their children for all to see and spoke about how successful they had been in their endeavours that year.

I participated in this charade every year, smiling and waving through gritted teeth. But things are very different when you are a stroke survivor. The noise created by other people can be very difficult to bear, so you want to be in familiar surroundings where you can easily move to another room if you get tired.

Family members should be willing to take this into consideration when discussing plans for Christmas, events or celebrations, and speak to the stroke survivor and their primary carer. Making plans without consulting the stroke survivor will only lead to disaster, as was the case in my situation.

Disputes hurt more when they are with a family member, sibling or parent, and I spent a very quiet and lonely Christmas with Asha.

I counted down the days to Ross' return and tried not to get stressed when things were in a complete shambles in the UK and another Coronavirus lockdown was imminent. Asha assured me everything would be okay and that we would make duas for him every night. The day Ross arrived we feasted like kings on Asha's famous biryani and lay in a food coma for several hours.

The family fallout had a very detrimental effect on the progress of my recovery. I lost more weight, dropping down to 43 kgs and I became very anxious at night. Lack of sleep made me lose focus during my physiotherapy sessions because I had no energy and my voice had become weaker. Even Joseph had to cancel a few physio sessions as I wasn't in the right frame of mind.

I cried so many rivers that even Justin Timberlake himself would have forgiven me, and I could feel myself sinking into depression. After countless chats with Ross, Asha and Joseph, I realised I needed to stop thinking about people who were upsetting me, focus on my health and find happiness again in life. The holidays reminded me that there were people who still loved me for who I was, and that was all that mattered.

I used to sing a lot when I was younger. I was in musicals in primary school, I joined a choir when I was in secondary school (with the sole purpose of meeting boys!) and in university I joined the Afro-Caribbean Harmonies, a singing group.

In 2013 I saw an advert in a weekly circular about singing and voice coaching. I always thought my voice was too deep and wanted to add power to it, especially when dealing with difficult clients. I met up with Tony Joett, a singing and voice coach, who helped me gain the confidence I was searching for. I thoroughly enjoyed the sessions and Joett got me out of my low alto comfort zone, and I was soon belting out songs like 'GoldFinger' by Shirley Bassey and 'SkyFall' by Adele.

One day I was in my bathroom showering when out of nowhere I started singing "On our way to freedom, we shall not be moved." I knew then that I needed to get to touch with Joett. Shortly afterwards I started working with him again. After just one session my spirits were lifted. Hearing my voice getting stronger each day has really helped me regain my confidence as I know that one day I will need to tell my story and talk to others going through similar recoveries.

Epilogue

"For what it's worth: it's never too late or, in my case, too early to be whoever you want to be. There's no time limit, stop whenever you want. You can change or stay the same, there are no rules to this thing. We can make the best or the worst of it. I hope you make the best of it. And I hope you see things that startle you. I hope you feel things you never felt before. I hope you meet people with a different point of view. I hope you live a life you're proud of. If you find that you're not, I hope you have the courage to start all over again."

- The Curious Case of Benjamin Button

There is no doubt that the last 4 months have been the most challenging months I have ever experienced. I was tested physically, emotionally and mentally so many times to the point where I wanted to give up.

What saved me was the constant reminder that God gave me a second chance. My life could have been taken away from me in an instant, I could have been confined to my bed or left in a vegetative state.

I had the opportunity in December 2020 of meeting Dr Kilalo Mjema, who was the ER doctor that attended to me when I first arrived in the Aga Khan Hospital a few short hours after my stroke. I had been looking out for her every time I went to the hospital for a consultation but she was always off duty on the days I visited.

Even though my recollection of that first visit to the ER was hazy, her face remained implanted in my memory. I was extremely happy and overcome with joy when I saw her again. I wanted to give her a massive hug but then I remembered the socially distanced circumstances that we were living in which meant that I had to contain myself.

I thanked her and her team for looking after me that day and for the amazing care I received at the hospital. I told Dr. Mjema one day I hoped to be able to work with her to help raise awareness of the preventative measures people can take to be able to detect the early signs of a stroke, rather than waiting until the last minute.

Every morning I wake up grateful to be alive and breathing and look forward to a day filled with new challenges which will make me stronger mentally and physically.

Talking to Joseph and Dr Praxeda has helped me accept what happened. In the early days I was in constant denial, waiting to wake up from what felt like a horrible nightmare. Whenever I would sit down to write, colour in or watch television I would lose myself in whatever I was doing, only to be reminded when I got up that I had had a stroke. This used to upset me a lot until Joseph told me that the feeling was normal since I didn't have any latent pain.

My fellow stroke survivor Sofia taught me so much about people and that you learn who you can and cannot rely on. There are those who genuinely care about your well being and wish to come and visit to encourage you, and others who want to see you so they can gossip to others about your condition. That is why it is so important to be careful who you surround yourself with. You control who does and does not visit you.

A lot of people fail to fully understand what a stroke is and think that the recovery process simply involves the rehabilitation of affected limbs. It is not like a broken toe or the flu, as my friend Jörg Potreck rightly pointed out.

My brain has had a total reboot as a result of the stroke. I had problems swallowing and eating, the entire right side of my body was weak and my speech impaired, so I had to learn many words again. I still get tired very easily even after completing simple tasks, and I some- times lose the ability to control my emotions, especially when I am tired, frustrated or feel that someone isn't listening to me.

I had to relearn a lot of simple motor skills that most people take for granted, such as tying shoe laces, doing up buttons and opening bottles of water. I even managed to put on some make up over the holidays using my left hand and attempted to put on my contact lenses on a different day. I struggled to get the right one out later and found out from the opticians that the right eye is still dry from the stroke and can't shut completely tight. That was why it was difficult to remove the contact as my eye isn't producing enough tears.

Thanks to encouragement and prayers from family and friends I have become stronger and more independent with the passing of each day. I can now shower and dress myself without supervision, make the bed in the mornings and get myself drinks from the fridge. I wash my own dishes after every meal and in the mornings if I wake up early and Ross is still tired, I will make my own breakfast and put away the dishes in the cupboards. I even recently ironed my first item of clothing using my right hand, being very careful not to burn myself. With more nerves and muscles becoming activated in my right hand I am now doing more with my hand. Every night before going to bed I try to massage my face using both hands, and even do the same for Ross if I sense he has had a long day and needs to relax. I am even able to write with right my hand. It isn't perfect but it is legible. And when I practise writing, I use both hands. Why? Because I can.

Dr Adebayo believes that I am ready to go back to work as soon as possible as reintegration into society will speed up my recovery. While I completely agree with his recommendation I would prefer to wait until I am ready, since he also said that I am my own doctor now.

I was a workaholic for almost 18 years. I lived and breathed work, thinking about it night and day, even when I went for a toilet break. I was so consumed by my job that I could often forget to eat, or eat very little because people always chose the wrong time to come see me. I never switched off and always thought about work even when I was on vacation.

I had been searching throughout my career for validation of my achievements to show my parents that their educational investment in me had not gone to waste. It was only recently that I realised that the validation had in fact been provided by my mentor, Dr Kapinga, who had been watching my legal career for many years.

I am learning to let go of the constant need for perfectionism, overworking and always being so hard on myself. The fact that I left my law firm in the hands of my team and have not checked on them even once shows that you have to let go of the reins once in a while.

I believe that there was a reason why the stroke happened my body was trying to tell me to slow down.

This forced time away from work is an opportunity for me to take it easy and give my brain the chance to heal properly. It might take 6 months or a year to fully heal. Anyone who attempts to try to rush me back to work sooner is inconsiderate and not looking out for what is best for me and my long term health.

I am still going through a lot of behavioural changes as a result of the reboot, which I need to learn to control. There have also been a few new changes which I am happy to embrace. In the past I always kept things buried inside for fear of confrontation, which would sometimes be detrimental to my well-being. One of the changes I am experiencing is that I speak out more about things that bother me. Some people are finding this hard to accept and would prefer the old, quieter Joy back.

I prayed for a better version of myself, someone who listens more, is empathetic, compassionate and is more attuned to other people's emotions. If other positive characteristics besides these arise that make me a happier person, why should I reject them? I embrace them.

My recovery is ongoing and I know that it will take time for me to be as fully functional as I can possibly be. I am learning to respect the limitations of my body and not push too hard, and I am working on becoming a better version of myself, ready to start over when the time is right.

Acknowledgments

This story would not have been possible without the hard work, support and love of the following people, to whom I owe my life and I am eternally grateful for my successful recovery.

The emergency doctors and nurses at Agha Khan Hospital who attended to me when I first arrived at the hospital. Dr. Phillip Adebayo, his team, Mama Naaz and all the nurses and orderlies at the Pavilion. The dietician Rozina Ratansi who has been working closely with my family to help with my weight gain post stroke. Dr. Eric Aris for introducing me to the Tanzania Stroke Association, which I look forward to being a part of once I am back on my feet. PT. Joseph Kisima for his friendship, for giving me hope in times of despair, his counsel and for teaching me how to be mobile again. Dr Praxeda Swai made me whole again and helped me realise the importance of mental health, and that sometimes you need to talk to a professional who will not judge you and will give you invaluable and impartial advice.

My father George Hadji Alliy and my oldest sister Lulu Alliy. Thank you for all the financial support that you provided during the earlier stages of my recovery and the support you provided Ross in managing my household and looking after me.

I cannot thank my brothers Mbwana and Mohamed Alliy enough for all their support. The maturity that they have shown and the way they have both handled matters has been exemplary. They listened to me, offered solutions to help create a more peaceful environment and tried their best to protect me as much as they could.

Thank you Araf Sykes for looking after my sister all this time. I can only imagine what she must have been going through at times, and I appreciate your patience and understanding.

My nephew Alijah Sykes who is one of kindest souls I have met. His smile brightens up the room, his endless hugs are full of warmth and love and he always made sure that "Tee" was not alone, offering me his old Dora the Explorer as a teddy bear to comfort me. I will never forget our discussions and alone time when we both took turns to read out loud to each other, in order to help strengthen my throat muscles.

My cousin Asha Mtindo is a godsend. I wouldn't have made it through the three weeks when Ross was away if it were not for her. She knows what I went through during that period, the amount of pain I suffered and how lonely I was. She kept my hopes up and binged on Netflix with me, and even started working out. If I can't do it right now I might as well do it vicariously.

Ross Methven has been my guardian angel ever since I lost my mother. He rescued me at a time when I had lost all hope of ever being happy again, and showed me how to live. Six years later he not only saved my life but went to hell and back with me. Ross puts up with my frustrating outbursts, always reminds me how far I have come whenever I feel discouraged, and has done so much more for me than I could have possibly imagined. Ross always used to say that he would be there for me no matter what and I used to think it was just empty words. I know now without a shadow of doubt that he meant every word.

Ross' parents Alastair and Anne Methven, his brother Niall and daughter Leah have been extremely supportive right from day 1. Although they are miles away in Edinburgh, their endless love and daily contact with Ross helped him stay sane especially during the sleepless nights.

The Novita Law team Flora Wamala, Agnella Mrope and Elizabeth Mwase rose to the challenge of manning the office on their own during this difficult period. I have the utmost confidence in their ability to hold the fort until I return and I am proud of the women that they have become.

Geofrey Danda, who helped the Novita Law team continue to manage the accounting side of the business during my absence.

Dr Wilbert Kapinga for being my mentor, for always there when I have a legal question, for teaching me how to become a trusted advisor and for being like an uncle to me.

Lucy Henry Sondo and Sofia-Magdalene Karlsson are two amazing women whose inspiring stories about stroke survival have kept me going through many dark days.

Family friends Triza Shinganya, Neema Hellela Charafeddine, Benedict Mponzi and Donald Galinoma for keeping my secret until I was ready to share it with the world. My adopted mother and auntie Grace Hellela for always being there for me. Her wise counsel has helped me get through many tough times and I am grateful to her children for sharing their mother with me.

Ross and I were unable to take up Peter Kasanda's generous offer to use his boat on the day the stroke happened.

Peter and I have been good friends for years, he always sent clients my way and kept in regular contact with Ross. When Ross' visa was about to run out, Peter put Ross in contact with immigration officials who helped him extend it.

Ex colleagues Jacktone Koyuji, Lotus Menezes, and Paul Bujingo who were there for me especially during the early days when I needed a lot of support and encouragement. Paul taught me a lot about letting go and that there is more to life than work.

My ex colleague Bart Wilm and his friend Sven Verboon have both been incredibly supportive over the years, and even more so when they heard about the stroke. They have both been truly amazing, listened to my story and challenges without judgement and even surprised me with flowers on my birthday.

My friends Sanaipei Ntimama, Fanny Nyembe, Nyaba Massinde, Nshesheye Msinjili Priebe, Alesumaniswa Maletmena Grossman, Sarah Hudson, Japhet and Joseph Kaseba, Hellen Michael, Aisha Sykes, Caroline Boswell, Mahbib Jemadari, Paul Muthaura, Rehema Ngamilo, Amish Shapriya, Valerie Vaz, Rebecca Young and Alison Grieve have all been amazing. Each one had their own unique way of encouraging, consoling and making sure I always had someone to talk to. This condition can break your soul if you let it, sinking you into an abyss of depression. I am so grateful to have friends that are making sure that will not happen to me.

Thank you Hellen Michael for coming up with the book title. You told me from day one that I would emerge from this experience wiser and stronger, and would use my voice to make sure I was heard.

Ross' team at work sent us a lovely card wishing me a speedy recovery, and rallied to manage the division during his absence. His colleague Trish Holt and her family have also been very supportive, sending the lovely get well drawings and heartfelt messages over the holidays.

His colleague David Brear was also very understanding and supportive especially when he was unable to work and look after me at the same time.

Ross' friends Steve Farquhar, Donald Hughes, Colin Ballantyne, Lindsay and Phil Gripton, Barry Shepherd, Gregor McKelvie, Jeff Tjissen, Alex Woodhouse, Roland Inglis, Ricky Hough, Tom Evans, Robbie Denoon and Mark Pavan sent me numerous get well wishes and provided him with welcome support.

The ladies of Glow Hair and Nails Salon were there to organise home visits when my hair felt like a bird's nest. My mother always made sure she looked good and took care of her skin, even when she was in the hospital, and it looks like I definitely inherited that trait from her.

Thanks to Inessa Hadjivayanis and her sister Dr. Ida Hadjivayanis. They always ask for updates and celebrate the small wins in my progress. They have been my cheerleaders even since they found out about the stroke. Inessa and Ida who work at the School of African and Oriental Studies have also been kind enough to help me translate my story into Kiswahili so I can reach a larger audience.

Thank you Tony Joett for taking me on as a challenge. I leave every session with a full heart knowing the hard work that we put in is helping to rebuild my confidence and make my voice stronger. I will share your tips on how to retain youthful looks with others.

And a special thank you to Dr Wilbert Kapinga, Ross Methven, Mohamed Alliy and PT. Joseph Kisima for reading early manuscripts, checking for grammatical errors and for their constructive comments.

Joy Hadji Alliy
joy.stroke.survivor@gmail.com
Dar es Salaam
February 2021

Printed in Great Britain
by Amazon

66623971R00071